Essential Oils for Bronchitis

Essential Oil Recipes for
Bronchitis
for Diffusers, Roller Bottles,
Inhalers & more.

Rica V. Gadi

Printed in the United States of America

First Printing, 2019

ISBN: 9781086065046

http://eorecipes.net

This book is dedicated to all the strong people who are taking responsibility for your own well being and doing something to be better.

All my heartfelt gratitude to the following people: my mom Ruby Jane, you have made me everything I am today; my dad Nestor-- my eternal, my angel, and the source of my perseverance; Mommyling, my spiritual guide ; Ria & Joe, the true witnesses of my transformation and my foundation pillars; Ellie Jane, the sparkle of our eyes;

Juan, thanks for always encouraging me to push harder - you are my ONE; Rocco & Radha, my reason for everything.

The Love of my family and friends is the fountain of inspiration that never runs dry. Thank you for constantly inspiring me, motivating me, and loving me unconditionally.

This book will never be complete without the help of my trusted and talented friends the #NOWsuperstars and my #oilbularya friends

Blending Essential Oils to use for a very specific reason has become very popular in recent years. There are several reasons why this is so. Blending EOs is basically about inhaling - as it has been proven that aromas have the ability to trigger feelings, emotions and personal memories.

With this in mind, it is obvious that everyone is unique when it comes to what triggers your senses. It all boils down to personal preference for the aroma to trigger what you want to unleash. Everyone is different and we all connect to the aroma differently, so what might work for one might not work for another person.

Of course, we also want the blend we personalize to be therapeutic. This is the best reason why to blend essential oils. We want the blend we create to help us with a very specific emotion or physical condition. As much as smelling good is important in a blend, it is more important that we blend oils that are not only pleasing to the smell but also produces the therapeutic effect we are after.

Then you have to think about contraindications. Making sure the blend you create is safe to use.

I suggest that before blending find out if the oils you are using is safe for a condition you may have example, if you are pregnant, or have specific allergies. Consult your physician prior to moving forward.

The recipes I have in this book is a compilation of what has proven to work and favored by hundreds of EO enthusiasts. It takes out the guesswork to get you started.

Again, we urge you to read the recipes and make sure that this is safe for you to try.

The book is very specific to a physical and emotional condition. There are several recipes here because you might want to rotate and you may like one and not the other. There is also a variety of applications. Some of us prefer to diffuse, some to make roller bottles, and others to create inhalers and sprays.

I hope you enjoy this compilation, feel free to use the notes section and jot down your fave blends. There is a wonderful world of EO blending - this is just the beginning.

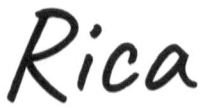

Bronchitis is a condition of the lungs wherein the bronchial tubes get inflamed. The bronchial tube is the airway to the lungs and when it gets inflamed, its inner lining swells and gets thicker; this narrows the airway and causes strain and blockage which results in symptoms such as a cough, shortness of breath, tightening in the chest, fatigue and wheezing. It is typically caused by viruses common to those that bring colds and flu. Bad habits such as cigarette smoking are also another cause of bronchitis due to the intake of toxic gases into the lungs. There are two main types of bronchitis, namely, chronic and acute bronchitis.

When the condition becomes chronic, ongoing medical treatment and regular visits to the doctor must be made to monitor the condition. Bronchitis can sometimes lead to pneumonia if not treated properly and not given enough attention. The body is already exposed to the virus and symptoms can escalate to a point where coughing can be so terrible that it brings up blood or mucus that is dark or thick. When symptoms last more than 3 weeks that is already a sign to get further help from the doctor.

Like plenty of diseases, there are plenty of alternative ways to reduce its symptoms to help while you recover. There is plenty of pain relief medicine that can be taken for physical ailments and for diseases like bronchitis, there are antibiotics, flu and cough medicine. There are also natural home remedies that can be done to help soothe the pain. When a cough is dry and painful during the first stages of bronchitis, using essential oils can help provide relief.

This is done through a diffused mixture of essential oils that can be inhaled for relief. A few examples of essential oils that can help bronchitis is eucalyptus dives oil, spike lavender oil, cedarwood oil, or frankincense oil. They provide antispasmodic and expectorant properties. There are also essential oils that can be applied topically and used as a chest rub; these are balsam fir, that can be calming and also has antimicrobial properties, and ginger oil that can help warm the body.

Table of Contents

Best Essential Oils for Bronchitis

There are a lot of different facets of human health, and maintaining a healthy life in each of them is incredibly important for anyone. Your respiratory system is one of the most vital components of your body, and when problems with breathing arise it can have a negative impact on every aspect of your life.

One such problem that could occur is bronchitis. It may not be as dangerous as some of the other lung and respiratory related problems; it can still have a very dramatic impact on your well-being. Luckily, it's something that can be controlled and managed effectively. By talking to your medical professional and charting out a plan for recovery, bronchitis can almost always be overcome.

Modern medicine and certain medications can be instrumental in making recovery come about more easily, using natural treatments like essential oils for bronchitis is something that's worth taking a look at as well.

1. Cinnamon has a long history not only as a wonderful spice for pastries but as a natural medicine too. Cinnamon essential oil increases circulation, bringing immune system cells to the lungs to clear respiratory ailments. It reduces inflammation in the bronchial tubes and fights viruses as well. Another good overall essential oil for the respiratory system, this essential oil helps reduce excess mucous, eases throat pain, and stimulates the immune system. Because cinnamon essential oil can be taken internally in small quantities, you can use it in teas, homemade cough syrup, and gargles.

2. Sage acquired its name by being regularly used by the Ancient Greeks to fight illnesses. Greek sage contains a high percentage of cineole like eucalyptus, and it is an anti-inflammatory, antibacterial, antiviral, and antiseptic. Be careful with this essential oil if you have low blood pressure, and avoid it during pregnancy. In small doses, this oil works wonders for most people to ease the symptoms of bronchitis.

3. Frankincense essential oil is known to reduce inflammation and pain, and because it soothes coughs and reduces phlegm, it's perfect for bronchitis sufferers. Frankincense calms the throat and nasal passages, and it is good to have on hand for allergies and asthma too. Frankincense is so effective that just a few drops inhaled from a handkerchief can provide relief from a multitude of symptoms.

4. The fresh, pine-like scent of rosemary essential oil makes it perfect for diffusion and other inhalation delivery routes when you have bronchitis. It opens all the breathing passages and fights resistant bacteria. Rosemary essential oil should be on your list for coughs, colds, bronchitis, sinusitis, and asthma. (Stay away from rosemary, however, if you have epilepsy or high blood pressure or if you are pregnant.

5. Peppermint essential oil common herb contains menthol. Many people use this essential oil for relief of congestion, although there is a lack of evidence that it actually helps. A study concluded that the inhalation of menthol does not actually relieve symptoms, but people who inhale it feel better anyway.

6. Lavender essential oil helps your asthma symptoms. One studyTrusted Source indicates that lavender oil inhalation inhibited airway resistance caused by bronchial asthma.

7. Tea Tree essential oil as Melaleuca. Most famous for its antimicrobial elements, tea tree essential oil fights yeast, fungi, and bacteria, even those that may be resistant to most antibiotics. Tea tree essential oil helps reduce inflammation, so it is perfect for bronchitis, where the bronchial tubes become swollen. It also eases a stuffy nose, reduces a cough, and combats sinusitis.

8. Eucalyptus essential oil as Melaleuca. Most famous for its antimicrobial elements, tea tree essential oil fights yeast, fungi, and bacteria, even those that may be resistant to most antibiotics. Tea tree essential oil helps reduce inflammation, so it is perfect for bronchitis, where the bronchial tubes become swollen. It also eases a stuffy nose, reduces a cough, and combats sinusitis.

9. Balsam fir essential oil is the right one for your recipes. It dries mucous, calms those embarrassing and choking coughing fits, and fights bacteria as well. Balsam fir essential oil supports your overall respiratory health so that you can breathe easier sooner.

10. Clove essential oil is an anti-inflammatory, and thus another good oil to fight bronchitis symptoms. Able to be taken internally like cinnamon, clove essential oil has multiple antimicrobial effects, combatting both bacteria and viruses. Its soothing, warmth makes it ideal for a cough and sore throat recipes.

11. An expectorant, **oregano essential oil** is another good choice to loosen phlegm and calms the wet cough that can accompany bronchitis. It is also an antiviral, antibacterial, and antifungal essential oil. If that weren't enough, oregano essential oil reduces respiratory inflammation and acts as an antioxidant, ridding the body of free radicals that can do cellular damage.

12. Thyme essential oil should be an ingredient in your bronchitis preparations. This essential oil is well studied as an antibacterial, although it is also beneficial for colds and flu. Thyme essential oil offers your immune system general support too so that you can recover faster from any temporary respiratory illness.

The Blending Process

These EOs are categorized by aromas, and EOs from the same group usually blend fantastically together.

- Floral – Lavender, Geranium, Jasmine
- Woodsy – Pine, Cedarwood
- Earthy – Vetiver, Patchouli
- Herbaceous – Marjoram, Rosemary, Basil
- Minty – Peppermint, Spearmint, Wintergreen
- Medicinal – Eucalyptus, Frankincense, Melaleuca
- Spicy – Pepper, Clove, Cinnamon
- Oriental – Ginger, Patchouli
- Citrus – Wild Orange, Lemon, Lime

Select oils that will give you with the health benefits you are looking to remedy. For increased energy choose: Grapefruit, Lemon, Orange, or Citrus. For Calming and Relaxation choose: Lavender, Cedarwood, or Chamomile. You are encouraged to experiment and play with your oils to see which blends work for you.

TIPS:

- Combine Floral EOs with Woodsy, Spicy and Citrus aromas
- Minty EOs with Woodsy, Earthy, Herbaceous and Citrus aromas
- Earthy EOs with Woodsy and Minty aromas
- Citrus EOs with Floral, Woodsy, Minty, Spicy and Oriental aromas

Diffuse

Diffusing Essential Oils is the safest
method to enjoy Essential Oils
without the risk of an allergic reaction.

Diffusing Essential Oils
Some Tidbits You Need To Know

Our sense of smell is one of our most powerful senses, and as you have noticed in your own experience that some scents affect your more positively in your minds than others. The body contains over 1,000 receptors for smell—way more receptors than for any of our other senses.

Diffusion Essential Oils means the process vaporizes oils into the air by releasing tiny amounts into the air. Inhalation is totally safe and is super low risk. Chances of any EO rising to dangerous levels while diffusion is slim to none.

Diffusing Essential Oils around newborns, babies, young children, pregnant or nursing women, and pets should be done with caution. Read up on safety.

It is advisable that Diffusing Essential Oils for only about 15-30 minutes at a time to be most effective. NEVER leave your diffuser on overnight. Make sure your diffuser is filled with the right amount of water and you understand the operating directions.

While diffusing essential oils, be sure that your space has great ventilation. Crack a window open if the scent becomes strong.

Never add Carrier Oils to your diffuser. This may cause your diffuser to malfunction. Clean your diffuser at least 3 times a week with warm water and natural soap to ensure the diffuser is well maintained and bacteria and mold does not accumulate.

Diffusing Essential Oils Basic Guidelines

Just a few things you need to know and prepare before getting started Diffusing Essential Oils.

Things you need:
Ultrasonic Oil Diffuser
Essential Oils
Water

Just follow the number of drops in the recipe, drop on to an oil diffuser and fill the rest with water.

All diffusers are different and will have its own water minimum and maximum level. Read the diffuser instruction before use.

Ideally, it is best to diffuse for 15-30 minutes and turn off the diffuser. The effect should be good for at least 2-3 hours. Turn your diffuser back on after 3 hours to reinforce oil diffusing effects.

It is not advisable to use EO in humidifiers.

These are not made to release EOS

Diffuser Recipes

Here's a thought for you:

You may be wondering how aroma can simply eliminate symptoms. There's a simple answer to this : Aroma is simply a by-product of diffusing. It's the added benefit but in reality the real benefit comes from the air we breathe and how the body easily absorbs the essential oils released into the air. It works 2 ways, not only does it improve the air quality you breath by disinfecting and eliminating pollutants it also allows your glands to absorb the healing elements of the EOs released in the air molecules,

So here are a few recipes that can help you manage symptoms and actual issues regarding the matter :

6 drops Clary Sage
4 drops Fir Needle
2 drops Lavender

----

2 drops Eucalyptus
1 drop Lemon
2 drops Peppermint

----

4 drops Eucalyptus
4 drops Peppermint

----

2 drops RC

2 drops Peppermint

----

5 drops Eucalyptus
2 drops Lemon

----

2 drops Lemon
2 drops Lavender
2 drops Peppermint

----

4 drops Frankincense
3 drops RC or Eucalyptus

----

1 drop Bergamot
1 drop Patchouli
1 drop Ylang Ylang

----

2 drops Lemon
2 drops Eucalyptus
2 drops Rosemary
1 drop Thyme

1 drops Lavender
2 drops Peppermint
2 drops Thyme
3 drops Eucalyptus

----

2 drops Rosemary
2 drops Pine
2 drops Marjoram
1 drop Lemon

----

3 drops Lemon
3 drops Scotch Pine
3 drops Lavender
1 drop Peppermint

----

3 drops Juniper Berry
4 drops Rosemary
4 drops Frankincense

----

4 drops Cypress
6 drops Grapefruit

3-5 drops Rosemary
2 drops Thyme
1 drop Peppermint
----

5 drops Cedarwood
4 drops Lavender
1 drop Chamomile
1 drop Eucalyptus (optional)

----

3 drops Pine or Cedarwood
3 drops Lavender
2 drops Eucalyptus
1 drop Lemon

----

2 drops Frankincense
2 drops Orange
1 drop Eucalyptus

3 drops Peppermint
3 drops Lemon
3 drops Eucalyptus

----

2 drops Oregano
2 drops Tea Tree
2 drops Peppermint
2 drops Lavender
2 drops Lemon

----

3 drops Tea Tree
2 drops Lavender
2 drops Peppermint

----

4 drops Lavender
4 drops Peppermint
2 drops Frankincense
2 drops Basil

----

3 drops Eucalyptus
3 drops Peppermint
3 drops Rosemary

Roll

Essential Oil Roller Bottles is the easiest method to enjoy Essential Oils Anywhere and Whenever.

Blending Essential Oils in a Roller Bottle
Some Tidbits You Need To Know

Essential Oils are usually super concentrated and too hard to measure how much to actually put straight from the bottle.

Roller bottles are a way that you are able to create blends ready to use with the right dilution. It allows your EO to last longer.

It also makes it easier to apply exactly where you want to target without getting it all over the place.

It is handy and easy to carry in your purse, ready to use at any time you want to.

I like to apply EOs at the bottom of the feet for many reasons. Our feet have bigger pores than any other skin in our bodies. this means that they are able to suck in the therapeutic compounds in our blend into the bloodstream faster than any other parts of the body. Imagine comparing a normal straw to an oversized straw and how much more you can suck in with the latter. This is how the soles of our feet is compared to the rest of the skin in our bodies.

The skin on our feet is also less sensitive and is designed to withstand some abuse. The risk of having an irritation from EOS is less likely to happen when applied on the feet.

The feet don't have the glands that act as a barrier. Sebaceous glands are glands in our skin that produces an oily substance called Sebum, for the purpose of lubricating and waterproofing the skin. Since this is oil and if you put oil on top of oil, it can act as a barrier or it may slow down penetration.

The feet and palms of our hands are the only skin that don't have these, so it is ideal to apply Essential Oils to the feet for maximum penetration.

Now, it would be hard to apply oils directly and very messy, right? Roller bottles make it super easy and convenient to roll the EOs at the bottom of our feet.

Carrier Oils Info

Carrier oils are vegetable-based oils with their own healing properties that dilute essential oils used to help carry the EOs into the skin.

Essential oils are highly concentrated and could evaporate very quickly. The carrier oil is mixed with the essential oil so it could penetrate the skin before it actually evaporates. Although EOs are oils, it is actually not that oily. When mixed with a carrier oil, it allows you to have more of the essential oil into your skin without wasting EOS to evaporate, making the healing properties of the EO strong and more effective.

There are also Essential oils that are too strong to apply directly to the skin and may cause damage, so it is important to dilute them with a carrier oil.

Never add Carrier Oils to your diffuser. This may cause your diffuser to malfunction. Clean your diffuser at least 3 times a week with warm water and natural soap to ensure the diffuser is well maintained and bacteria and mold does not accumulate.

Carrier Oils

There are a lot of different carrier oils that you can use with EOs to dilute them in a roller bottle.

To name a few :

Almond Oil - moisturizing and stays liquid at room temperature. Do not use if you are allergic to nuts.

Apricot Kernel Oil - moisturizing and suitable for sensitive skin or kids. It is super gentle on the skin.

Avocado Oil - moisturizing and suitable for sensitive and damaged skin. Perfect for skin problems.Can be mixed with other carrier oils

Castor Oil - with antibacterial, antiviral and antifungal properties, use topically to eliminate pain and relieve skin irritation.

Coconut Oil - its antibacterial, antiviral and antifungal properties it is the best and most versatile for skin care. The skin absorbs this very quickly. It solidifies in room temp and may still have a slight coconut oil aroma in it - but you can get fractionated coconut oil to eliminate the 2 challenges above.

Grapeseed Oil - not just for cooking but also great for topical application on the skin.

Jojoba Oil - one of my faves for skin care blends. This oil is the closest to our natural oil our skin produces to it is absorbed easily without being oily. Also amazing for massage oil blends.

Olive Oil - this is the oil for herb type oils. mostly used for cooking but can also be applied to the skin but would need to be blended with a carrier oil that is mild and absorb well with the skin.

Rosehip Seed Oil - super good for deep moisturizing or skin irritations. This oil has a high content of antioxidants and helps remedy dry, scarred and wounded skin.

Recommended Roller Bottle Dilution Guide

RECOMMENDED ROLL-ON BOTTLE DILUTION AMOUNTS

5 ml (1/6 oz.) Roll-on Bottle = ~100 drops (1tsp.)
10 ml (1/3 oz.) Roll-on Bottle = ~200 drops (2 tsp.)
30 ml. (1 oz.) Roll-on Bottle = ~600 drops (6 tsp.)

Roll-on Size	5 ml	10 ml	30 ml	Add EO drops to roll-on, then fill with carrier oil.	
Essential Oil Drops	1	2	6	1%	Dilution Percentage
	2	4	12	2%	
	3	6	18	3%	
	5	10	30	5%	
	10	20	60	10%	
	20	40	120	20%	
	25	50	150	25%	
	50	100	300	50%	

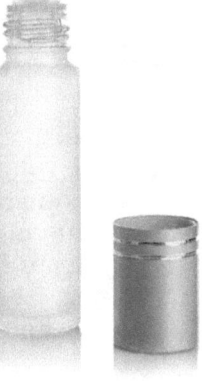

General Guidelines:
Birth to 12 months = .3-.5% dilution
1-5 years = 1.5-3% dilution
6-11 years = 1.5-5% dilution
12-17 years = 1.5-20% dilution
18 years and older = 1.5% dilution-Neat (no dilution)
Elderly or Sensitive Skin = 1-3% dilution
Daily Use = 2-5% dilution
Short Term Use = 10-25% dilution
Local Skin or Systemic Issues = 50% dilution-Neat

These are general guidelines suggestions--not absolute rules--based on traditional aromatheraphy practice.
(Kurt Schnaubelt PhD, Valerie Worwood, Robert Tisserand)

Dilution Basics:

How much you dilute your EO depends on different factors such as weight, sensitivity, health conditions, EOs that are blended in or how long that blend has been used for. There is never an absolute dilution rule, it is you who knows about your level and tolerance. I feel that it is best to start with a higher dilution percentage and increase EO drops over time.

To make sure your EO is safe, make sure that the oils you use are therapeutic grade and do your research on the source and extraction methods used to produce the oils.

Roller Bottle Blending Order

I normally just start with dropping the drops of oil into the **10mL roller bottle**, then adding the carrier oil up until the shoulder of the bottle. Capping the bottle off with the roller and the bottle cap. Instead of shaking the bottle, i like to roll the bottle between my palms first for a minute or 2 for blending, then finishing it off with a few shakes.

NOTE: All recipes in this book is for a 10mL Roller Bottle. If you have a bigger or smaller roller bottle, adjust the number of EO drops based on the size of your bottle.

Roller Bottle Recipes

5 drops Onguard
5 drops Oregano
5 drops Lemon

----

9 drops Respiratory Blend
7 drops Lime

----

5 drops Eucalyptus
3 drops Frankincense
2 drops Lemon

----

10 drops Breathe
5 drops Lime

----

10 drops Respiratory Blend
5 drops Eucalyptus
5 drops Frankincense

----

4 drops Lemon
4 drops Peppermint
2 drops Frankincense

----

6 drops RC
4 drops Lemon
4 drops Purification
2 drops Thyme
----

2 drops Palo Santo
4 drops Myrrh
5 drops Clove
6 drops Ravensara

----

6 drops of Lavender
4 drops of Rosemary
3 drops of Peppermint
2 drops of Eucalyptus

----

6 drops Eucalyptus
3 drops May Chang
4 drops Black Pepper
2 drops Peppermint
2 drops Rosemary

----

2 drops Oregano
2 drops Melaleuca
2 drops Lemon
2 drops Frankincense
2 drops Cinnamon

----

8 drops Cypress
4 drops Frankincense
4 drops Orange

----

8 drops Cedarwood
8 drops Eucalyptus
2 drops Roman Chamomile

----

10 drops Breathe
5 drops Eucalyptus

----

6 drop Cardamom
6 drop Frankincense
----

2 drops Oregano
2 drops Tea Tree
2 drops Lemon
2 drops Frankincense
2 drops Cinnamon

----

4 drops Peppermint
2 drops Eucalyptus
2 drops Lemon

----

2 drops Lemon
6 drops Lavender
2 drops Peppermint

----

5 drops Eucalyptus Radiata
2 drops Eucalyptus Citriodora
2 drops Myrtle
2 drops Peppermint
2 drops Spruce
2 drops Ravintsara
2 drops Pine
2 drops Marjoram

----

5 drop Oregano
5 drop Thyme

Bonus Recipes

Bronchitis Rub

10 drops Breathe
5 drops Thyme
5 drops Wintergreen
5 drops Oregano
5 ml. Bottle

Bronchitis Massage Oil

2 tbsp Carrier Oil
6 drops Lemon
6 drops Peppermint
10 drops RC
3 drops Raven
2 drops Thieves

Nighttime Flu Relief

8 drops Lavender
6 drops Frankincense
6 drops Lemon
4 drops Eucalyptus
4 drops Tea Tree
4 drops Peppermint
4 drops Roman Chamomile

Throat Tickle Tamer

2 drops Myrrh
2 drops Lemon
2 drops Cassia
1 tbsp Coconut oil
1 tbsp Raw honey

DIY Cough Rub

1/4 cup Coconut Oil
1/4 cup Shea Butter or Beeswax
20 drops Eucalyptus
5 drops Tea tree
5 drops Lavender
5 drops Lemon
5 drops Peppermint

Inhale

Essential Oil Inhalers are the most convenient way to enjoy Essential Oils Anywhere and Whenever.

Essential Oil Inhalers give you quick and easy access to the vast therapeutic benefits of essential oils.

Blending Essential Oils in an Inhaler
Some Tidbits You Need To Know

EO Inhalers or aroma sticks are compact tubes, with a cotton wick inside and a protective cover, to lock the aroma within.

Your preferred blend of essential oils is absorbed by the cotton wick, and safely enclosed in a tube that fits inside of the cover. The cover is easily removed for access to the tube to breathe in the aroma. Usually lasts about 3 months, depending on the oil blend used.

I absolutely love these because they encourage me to take a moment during super stressful moments, and just breathe.

It is in times of stress when our breathing patterns often change and taking deep breaths promote a feeling of calm and inner peace. Breath work combined with visualization plus a relaxing inhaler, can offer relief to symptoms of stress and help your body to come back to the state of homeostasis.

Aroma Sticks can be carried in your tiny purse, even compact enough to fit in your pocket. You can enjoy your favorite EOs anywhere and you can use them with discretion.

I love diffusing, and do all the time but not everyone in my space may enjoy the scents I enjoy or they may not benefit from the therapeutic benefits of the EOs I am diffusing - so the inhaler is one way to not only enjoy my choice of blends but to keep in personal not affecting everyone else around me.

Inhalers not only benefits me but also keep those around me safe in case the oils I want to blend may pose a risk to those around me who may have a health issue not advised to be exposed to my choice EOs/

When making Aroma Sticks, You may use your chosen EOs at 100% Concentration.

Inhaler Basic Guidelines

Breathe in slow and deep to absorb the EO molecules directly into your olfactory system.

Inhalers are super easy to use. You just remove the cap and inhale from the inhaler tube, count 1 to 5 slowly as you inhale. The EO molecules get drawn into our bloodstream through our nasal cavity and gets delivered throughout our entire body.

Simple to use, easy to cary, portable and compact. You never have to be without your favorite blends, ever.

Inhaler Blending Basics

Inhalers are super easy and simple to make.

All you need is an inhaler set which consist of the following:

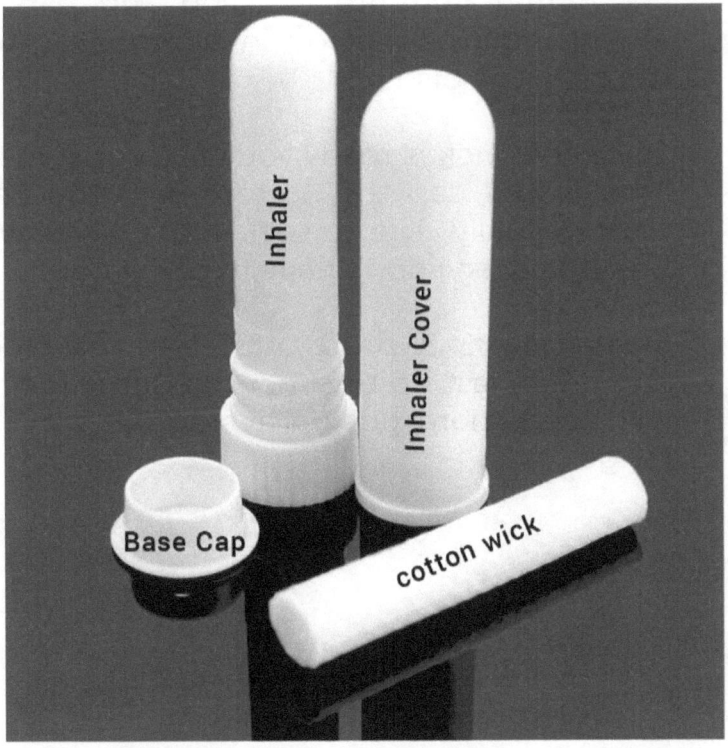

Inhaler, Inhaler Cover, Base Cap and Cotton Wick.

You will need your Essential Oils.

I like to use a pipette for precision and a small petri dish so I can see the oil.

Blending is super easy, just combine the drops and swirl it around in the petri dish and when you are satisfied you can go ahead and drop the cotton wick to absorb all the oil in the dish.

Once the wick is ready you can drop it in the inhaler and cap the bottom with the Base Cap. I usually like to secure the cover with the inhaler so I don't have to do it later.

I usually us 15-20 drops of EO total in a recipe and it can last up to 3 months. Some recipes will need more but on average it is in this range.

Inhaler Recipes

5-7 drops of Pine or Cedarwood
5-7 drops of Lavender
4 drops of Eucalyptus
1 drop of Lemon

----

5 drops Cedarwood
5 drops Lavender
5 drops Tea Tree

----

5 drops Pine
5 drops Lavender
4 drops Eucalyptus
1 drop Lemon

----

4 drops Peppermint
4 drops Lavender
4 drops Eucalyptus
2 drop Lemon
2 drops Rosemary

6-8 drops Peppermint
4-6 drops Eucalyptus
4-6 drops Rosemary

----

2 drops Peppermint
5 drops Thyme
8 drops Rosemary

----

6 drops Lavender
5 drops Frankincense
2 drops Peppermint
1 drop Oregano

----

3 drops Oregano
3 drops Tea tree
3 drops Lemon
3 drops Frankincense
3 drops Cinnamon leaf

----

5 drops Black Pepper
5 drops Frankincense
5 drops Black Spruce

----

5 drops Eucalyptus
5 drops Peppermint
5 drops Lemon

----

5 drops Lavender
5 drops Peppermint
5 drops Lemon

----

5 drops Cypress
5 drops Eucalyptus
5 drops Tea Tree

----

2 drops Oregano
2 drops Peppermint
2 drops Tea Tree
2 drops Lavender
2 drops Lemon

----

2 drops Eucalyptus
2 drops Patchouli
2 drops Peppermint

----

3 drops Eucalyptus
3 drops Thyme
3 drops Peppermint
3 drops Basil
3 drops Rosemary

----

3 drops Balsam Fir
2 drops Frankincense Carteri
2 drops Grapefruit Pink
1 drop Orange Sweet

----

6 drops of Eucalyptus
6 drops of Roman Chamomile

----

4 drops of Balsam Fir
6 drops of Roman Chamomile
10 drops of Frankincense

----

3 drops Geranium
2 drops Oregano
2 drops Cinnamon
1 Peppermint

----

3 drops Bergamot
3 drops Tea tree
2 drops Cinnamon
2 Peppermint

XX

Book Ordering

To order your copy / copies of

Essential Oils
for Bronchitis

please visit: **EOrecipes.net**

You can also check out other titles
available.

Bulk Pricing and
Affiliate Programs Available